"I Need Help"

"I Need Help"

A STROKE PATIENT'S PLEA

UNDERSTANDING
SIMPLIFIED MEDICAL TERMINOLOGY
AND ANATOMY
WITH EMPHASIS ON STROKE
(CEREBROVASCULAR ACCIDENT OR CVA)
INCLUDING SYMPTOMS
AND CONCRETE SUGGESTIONS
FOR PATIENTS AND CAREGIVERS

BY
HELEN UNDERWOOD, (RET.) R.N. (U.C.S.F.)
Certified Long-Term Care Ombudsman
1st Lt. Army Nurse Corps.
Accredited Record Technician
Certified In-service Educator
Director of Staff Development
Activity Coordinator
Medical Record and Nursing Consultant
California Community College Teaching Credential
(Health Services)

Blue Dolphin

Published by
Blue Dolphin Publishing, Inc.
P.O. Box 1908, Nevada City, CA 95959

ISBN: 0-931892-72-4

Library of Congress Cataloging-in-Publication Data
Underwood, Helen, 1914–
    I need help : a stroke patient's plea / by
Helen Underwood.
        p.   cm.
    ISBN 0-931892-72-4 : $8.95
    1. Cerebrovascular disease—Popular
works.   2. Aphasia—Popular works.
I. Title.
RC388.5U52 1991
616.8'1—dc20   91-27780
                                                    CIP

Basic Needs Illustrations by Sarah Poynter
Printed in the United States of America by
Blue Dolphin Press, Inc., Grass Valley, California

9   8   7   6   5   4   3   2   1

Table of Contents

Author's Note   7

Part I: Understanding Stroke   9
1. Definition of Stroke   11
2. Causes of Stroke   13
3. Symptoms of Stroke   16
4. Assisting the Paralyzed   18
5. Assisting the Aphasic   21
6. Suggestions in Summary   24

Part II: Understanding Geriatrics   29
    Introduction   30
7. The Acute Facility Versus
    the Extended Care Facility   31
8. Body Systems   37
    Skeletal System   37
    Muscular System   41
    Respiratory System   44
    Gastrointestinal System   48
    Cardiovascular (Circulatory) System   53
    Genitourinary System   58
    Nervous System   62
    Endocrine System   67
    Organs of Special Sense   71

9. Understanding Nuclear Medicine
    and Diagnostic Procedures   74

Part III: Understanding
        Medical Terminology   77
10. Medical Terminology   79
    Medical Abbreviations   81
    Prefixes   85
    Roots   89
    Suffixes   94

Part IV: Basic Needs Illustrations   97
11. Basic Needs Illustrations   99
    Pain/Itch   100
    Thirsty   101
    Hungry   102
    Turn over   103
    Bed up/down   104
    Bedpan   105
    Urinal   106
    Toilet   107
    Too hot   108
    Too cold   109
    Light off/on   110
    Brush teeth   111

Author's Note

THIS PUBLICATION IS WRITTEN TO EMPHASIZE the importance of better understanding and appropriate response to the *frustrations* experienced in problems of many patients, primarily paralysis and difficulties in communication in varying degrees (aphasia). As you read, *try to visualize yourself personally* in a similar situation, realizing that brain damage can occur at any age, at any time.

The suggestions herein have been accumulated by personal experience in caring for hundreds of such patients, as well as having taught many Nursing Assistants over the years.

In order to accurately understand the severe problems of stroke, one must relate on a personal level.

Just try to imagine both paralysis and aphasia: You wake up during the night in pain (and possibly some itching), and unable to communicate, let alone respond to either—even to turn over or change your position.

I relate most vividly to my mother's dilemma (massive stroke with almost total paralysis and aphasia and tunnel vision) when she could only respond by tears, and that only if one stood *directly* in front of her.

Less personal, but far more tragic, is my recollection of caring for two teenagers suffering from brain damage (motorcycle and automobile accidents) with paralysis and aphasia and basically no prospect of recovery to any extent.

I am deeply indebted to Solveig Crawford, RN, PHN, BS, and MA; Millie James, RN, PHN, and BHS; and my son, William H. Underwood, Registered Practicing Radiologic Technologist (specializing in MRI and CT scanning), for their time-consuming and very helpful editorial suggestions.

I hope this information will help both the caregiver and the patient in responding to the stroke patient's needs.

—H.U.

Part I

Understanding Stroke

Definition of Stroke
Causes of Stroke
Symptoms of Stroke
Assisting the Paralyzed Patient
Assisting the Aphasic
Suggestions in Summary

1

Definition of Stroke

STROKE, OR CEREBROVASCULAR ACCIDENT (CVA) is described as destruction of brain substance resulting from intracranial hemorrhage, thrombosis, or embolism which causes vascular insufficiency. In other words, an area of the brain does not receive the necessary blood because of a ruptured or blocked blood vessel. When oxygen and blood are cut off from a part of the brain, the cells in that part of the brain are damaged. How the patient is affected depends upon where the damage occurs. The stroke patient may have one-sided, both lower extremities and possibly trunk, or all four extremities, weakness or paralysis (inability to move), loss or diminished sensations of touch, memory, emotions, and/or aphasia (communication defect or loss of the power of expression by speech, writing, or signs, or understanding spoken or written language in varying degrees). Stroke has also been described as a sudden loss of feeling and movement of the body except for respiration. There are also "minor strokes" (fleeting and temporary with no structural damage).

The clinical picture of a stroke varies widely. It may be a violent attack in which the patient falls suddenly, deprived of motion and sense; however, the most frequent type is that in which there is variable defect in speech, motion, thought, vision, or sensation without loss of consciousness. In the latter case, some degree of recovery is almost always certain. The violent attack is usually caused by massive cerebral hemorrhage and the more mild attack is usually due to thrombosis. It is always important to keep in mind that almost all patients can be helped to some degree, even though the process can be extremely slow and requires much patience.

2
Causes of Stroke

THERE ARE THREE DIFFERENT EVENTS that result in a stroke.

1) *Cerebral Hemorrhage:* During the aging process the arteries in the brain degenerate and become brittle. In this event and if the blood pressure is also raised, the brittle arteries sometimes burst. Massive hemorrhage may even occur in the absence of hypertension. The site of the hemorrhage and also the extent of the hemorrhage will naturally determine the effect. The most common site is unfortunately that part of the brain where the motor nerves to the body are in a small space before passing down the spinal cord. In this event the motor impulses are cut off from the muscles of the face, arm, and leg on the side of the body affected. Because the motor nerves from one side of the brain cross to the opposite side before passing down the cord, hemorrhage on the right side of the brain is followed

by a left-sided paralysis and hemorrhage on the left side of the brain results in right-sided paralysis. Since the speech center in right-handed persons is on the left side of the brain, hemorrhage on the left side destroys the nerve fibers that go to the organs of speech, causing speechlessness or problems with speech (aphasia).

2) *Thrombosis:* The most common cause of strokes (around 50% of all cases) is caused by thrombosis (clot) which obstructs the extracerebral vessels, most likely the carotid in the neck and the vertebral artery. In these instances the symptoms can vary to a great extent depending on the site of the vessel that is blocked off and the size of the area of the brain affected. It sometimes takes several days for the neurological symptoms to develop. A stroke caused by thrombosis usually occurs while the patient is asleep or shortly after awakening in the morning.

3) *Cerebral Embolism:* The third cause of stroke is embolism of the smaller cerebral vessels within the brain. The embolism most often originates in the heart and then passes into the carotid artery

to the middle cerebral artery, resulting in paralysis which may be very extensive. Symptoms of this type of stroke come on very suddenly (within seconds) and with total absence of any warning. Stroke due to embolism may occur at any time of the day or night.

Symptoms of Stroke

L*OSS OF CONSCIOUSNESS:* Coma can occur immediately after the onset of a stroke. The length of the coma depends upon the severity and location of the problem. Vital signs are usually normal in a stroke, but when coma is present the temperature is often elevated with rapid pulse.

Headache, Nausea, Vomiting, and Convulsions: These symptoms can be present in varying degrees after the patient regains consciousness, the severity again being determined by the extent of the problem.

Paralysis: Paralysis is defined as loss or impairment of the ability to move parts of the body. The type of paralysis depends on whether the damage is to the central nervous system (as in stroke) or to the peripheral nervous system (a loss of power due to a lesion of the nervous mechanism between nucleus of origin and periphery). In stroke the paralysis usually causes some permanent disability; however, much can be done to rehabilitate the patient. Hemiplegia (common in stroke) is defined as paralysis of one side of the body; paraplegia is paralysis of the legs and possibly the lower trunk, and quadriplegia is paralysis of all four limbs.

Speech Disturbance: In a patient with severe stroke, one of the most frustrating problems is aphasia (disturbance or loss of ability to speak or write or comprehend another's speech, as previously described). The patient may have slurred speech and difficulty talking if the muscles of the face and mouth are affected. When facial paralysis is present the aphasia is sometimes complicated by drooping of the mouth and drooling of saliva. In motor aphasia the patient knows what he wants to say but can't say or write the words he wants to use. Please remember, though, that often he still is able to think, usually quite clearly. In sensory aphasia, the patient has inability to comprehend spoken or written language. There are also other variances of aphasia.

Other symptoms have previously been referred to under "Definition of Stroke."

4
Assisting the Paralyzed Patient

IN THE EVENT OF PARALYSIS a Physical Therapist is most usually consulted after initial evaluation by the physician. As stated previously, the motor impulses are cut off from the muscles of the face, arm, and leg on the side of the body affected, resulting in varying degrees of paralysis. Remember, hemorrhage on the right side of the brain is followed by left-sided problems and visa versa.

The most common type of paralysis in the stroke patient is hemiplegia—neuromuscular destruction of one side of the body (arm, face, leg), the facial paralysis complicating the communication problem.

It is extremely important that the Nursing Staff and other Caregivers (i.e. Home Nursing Aide and family) be totally involved in the problem of rehabilitation as set forth by the Physical Therapist. The person involved should be directly instructed by the Therapist, if at all possible, and be made aware of the importance of the procedures and the fact that harm could result if there is negligence or lack of continuity.

Physical Therapy, also known as Physiotherapy, is involved in physical restoration of affected parts (as in the hemiplegic stroke patient) and uses specific exercises and an activity program to encourage the highest level of physical fitness, also in emphasizing programs in areas of daily living. Physiotherapy is most commonly in the form of exercise and massage, although electrotherapy, heat, and radiation therapy are occasionally used.

In event of paralysis, decubitus (bed sore) is often a complication and is much easier prevented than cured. If the patient is unable to turn and/or is incontinent, the problem is even more complicated. Cleanliness and changing positions (sheets, pads, etc. in event of incontinence), at least every two hours, is mandatory especially if any reddened areas are observed.

Aside from the Caregiver's total understanding of the proper procedures for each case, as demonstrated by the Therapist, patient motivation is extremely important. Progress is usually very slow so the patient requires much encouragement by all persons involved. If at all possible, depending upon the patient's degree of understanding, he should be informed of the type of disability he suffers and reasons for the individual therapy.

5

Assisting the Aphasic Patient

AS DESCRIBED UNDER SYMPTOMS of the stroke patient, aphasia, or problem with communication, is extremely frustrating to the patient and all persons concerned. The disturbance can be either spoken or written and in varying degrees of severity.

The most important consideration in helping the aphasic patient is to consider how you yourself would feel if in a similar situation. Just try to imagine your reaction if you very suddenly, without any warning whatsoever, found that you could not speak, could not convey the fact that you were thirsty, hungry, unable to turn over or move a part of your body, needed to go to the bathroom, could not even describe any pain you might be feeling (location and extent), and basically had no understanding of what had happened to you. It is only in realizing all of this that you can be of major assistance to the patient.

It is also important to recognize that aphasia is very complex, as is the brain that has been affected. It is not uncommon for the aphasic to show anger, depression, sudden tears, emotional outbursts, etc. without any other apparent cause.

If the patient is aphasic but can communicate by pointing, or even by blinking or smiling, on the last pages of this book you will find pictures of basic needs to which your patient can refer. There will be additional needs as to particular patients, so you may wish to add to these illustrations. In a few isolated cases patients have been able to be understood if they are encouraged to point to letters of the alphabet in order to form words.

As indicated, prognosis in event of aphasia usually depends upon the severity of the problem. The following are the most likely possibilities:

1. When the patient has many physical problems, as well as aphasia, to a significant degree, the Nursing Home or Extended Care Facility will likely be the ultimate solution to follow-up care after Acute Care hospitalization. As described

later, there are, more recently, Acute Rehabilitation hospitals for specific patients.

2. Age and patient determination, as well as dedication of Caregiver, are also considerations in type of Long-Term Care.

3. After initial hospitalization, including evaluation by Physician, Speech Pathologist, Physical, Cardiopulmonary, and Occupational Therapists, with good potential, many times the patient can be maintained at home with supervision.

6
Suggestions in Summary

1. Encourage even the slightest effort the patient may make. Try to reassure that you *expect* him to improve—this will prevent him from giving up and not making further effort. Remember that even though the response may not be correct, there is at least an attempt which could well improve with time.

2. Do not talk to others in the patient's presence if the topic is at all negative. One can never be absolutely sure just how much your patient is understanding when he has no way of responding, and your main purpose is to encourage in any possible way so as to prevent your patient from giving up his endeavors. (This advice is also very important as pertains to a terminal patient, suffering from any disorder, as one can never be positive as to the true mental condition even if coma is seemingly evident.)

3. Do not hesitate to repeat your statements or questions slowly, giving time for the patient to absorb and attempt response—i.e., "Would you like some water?" "Water?" "Fruit Juice?" "Fruit Juice?".

4. Never belittle the patient by using abnormal language—i.e. childish tones. Even though he cannot speak or respond in any way, he most likely hears and understands almost anything you say. Assume by the way you yourself are communicating that this is true and your results will be much more encouraging.

5. Use short sentences and simple words so as to be more understandable in case he is having problems in concentrating. Speak somewhat slower and give him ample time to at least attempt a response even if only by facial expression.

6. When asking questions, accept head nods and also phrase the question so that it is appropriate for the patient to reply by using the most simple answer, such as just "Yes" or "No." If you ask him, "What kind of food would you like?" he

may not be able to respond, whereas if you say "Would you like some soup?" he could more easily respond.

7. Participation in any activity planned by family or Facility is of utmost importance whenever feasible. This is of great concern in relieving symptoms of depression which are inevitable in any disease of long term and much more so when communication is not possible.

8. In event the patient is trying to start a sentence, try to be very patient and allow him plenty of time to gather his thoughts. This is sometimes quite difficult but very essential, and your interference may discourage him from trying.

9. Use the pictures in the back of the book whenever appropriate, or cut pictures from magazines. If you are unsure of his desires, try pointing to the picture and ask him, "Is this what you want?" You might also ask him to repeat the word so that he might be able to tell you the next time.

10. There are several additional things you may wish to resort to in the event you cannot comprehend the problem:

a. You might say, "I don't understand. Did you mean that you _____?"

b. Ask him to try to say the same thing again, repeat his request back to him.

c. If he becomes quite frustrated, as often occurs, postpone the conversation temporarily but be sure that you tell him you will return and try again. In this event, be *sure* that you follow through with your promise.

d. If able to write, provide some paper and an easy to hold thick pen.

e. Keep hearing aid, glasses, and clock close at hand.

f. Place a call bell within reach.

g. If there are problems in swallowing, this indicates lack of muscle control or loss of feeling in the mouth is present. Give the patient small bites of food and liquid and instruct holding of breath while swallowing so that the food does not go down the trachea which could cause breathing problems.

h. A personal scrapbook of mementos and photographs of family, pets, etc. (things closest to the family) can be very useful.

i. Basically, experimentation is the key to becoming the most helpful. As previously explained, there are actually no two stroke patients who have exactly the same problems, either in motor or speech areas.

The family can be very informative in revealing the personality, type of employment, activity interests, etc., thereby giving you a background from which to explore. There are also some new highly scientific communication aids (i.e. voice synthesizers) that could be explored, perhaps through a Speech Therapist.

PART II

Understanding Geriatrics

Introduction

The Acute Facility Versus
the Extended Care Facility

Body Systems

Understanding Nuclear Medicine and
Diagnostic Procedures

INTRODUCTION

THERE IS AN EVER-GROWING NEED for well-informed medical and paramedical workers in the Extended Care Field due to tremendous expansion as longevity increases with current rapid strides and expertise in the medical field.

This part of the book is geared toward providing *basic* information to anyone entering the area of Gerontology and Rehabilitation, and as a refresher for those with previous experience.

There is emphasis on the basic differences between the Acute and the Extended Care Facility, not always clearly understood by either employee or patient. More recently Rehabilitation Hospitals have been developed (primarily stroke rehab.) with object of discharge to home within 4-6 weeks. These consist of a team of Physicians, Nurses, Physical, Occupational, Cardiopulmonary, Speech, and Recreational Therapists.

Many areas such as "Body Systems" and "Medical Terminology" (in Part III) are covered in simple, concise format, so that information will be readily available for future reference.

7

The Acute Facility Versus The Extended Care Facility

THE FOLLOWING IS A SIMPLIFIED DESCRIPTION of various nursing facilities—not strictly applicable to all, as state regulations change on occasion and vary according to size and needs.

1) **Acute Facilities** require a Hospital Administrator, Medical Directors, Director of Nursing Services and Assistant Director, Registered and some Licensed Vocational/Practical Nurses, Medical Record Department, Discharge Planner, Physical, Speech, Occupational, Cardiopulmonary Therapists, Emergency and Outpatient, Laboratory, X-ray, Surgery, Dietary, Pharmacy, Business, Housekeeping, Maintenance Departments, and other areas if indicated, as well as Certified Nursing Assistants. (N.A.s participate in a 150 hr. course of lecture and practical experience for certification in California.) Periodic inspections are made by the State Health Depart-

ments (as in all facilities) and staff meetings are held regularly. Upon discretion of the Physician/Surgeon, the Visiting Nurse Association or a Home Health Agency can make follow-up visits upon patient discharge to home or other facility. Outpatient care in acute facilities has rapidly increased in the past years, thereby including such surgical procedures as cataract removal and eliminating overnight stay.

2) Convalescent Hospitals and Nursing Centers (Extended Care) offer a continuation of nursing care, to include an Activity Coordinator, except on a much more limited scale as patients are obviously not in need of nearly as much nursing care and supervision. Utilization Review Committee meetings are held at regular intervals at which Medical, Nursing, and Record personnel evaluate charts to verify that patient needs and regulations are met as in acute facilities. Obviously far fewer departments are required than in Acute Care. Ombudsmen (individuals who have completed short courses in regulations) monitor problems and complaints of nursing homes and residential facilities under the authority of the

Older Americans' Act. The newer Rehabilitation Centers are also available for short-term stay after acute care.

3) Board and Care: These homes are usually small but must also meet strict health and safety requirements. Patients receive board and care with medications dispensed by a competent person, and an attendant in the building at all times.

4) Home: The ultimate goal is to rehabilitate the patient so that he may return home if at all possible. Home Health Care services are available intermittently or on a continual basis.

CONCLUSIONS

The patient obviously needs and receives more actual medical attention in the Acute Hospital, which in many cases creates a problem in that the patient and/or family often expects virtually the same of the Physician and Nursing Staff in the Extended Care Facility. Keep in mind the financial disparity that exists between the categories and the obvious need for keeping within the budget requirements. The patient will likely be paying a good deal less than the cost of Acute Facility care when transferring to Extended Care, and less in Board and Care as he improves and becomes more independent. Some of the other basic differences in Acute versus Extended Care are as follows:

Average length of stay in the Acute Facility can be a day or more, while Extended Care can expect a stay of undetermined length (exceptions of course would include the patient transferring from the Acute Facility for short-stay convalescence following major surgery, etc.).

In the Acute Facility the doctor sees his patient every day, whereas the doctor in the Extended Care Facility at present is not required to see his patient except monthly unless complications should arise. Physical, Occupational, Speech Therapy and the Cardiopulmonary Department are available as needed.

The Extended Care Facility has need for functions such as Activity Programs, Social Services, Mental Health, Community resources (i.e. volunteers, service clubs, etc.), as well as Therapies as individually ordered.

As you can see, there are many differences from Acute Facility to Extended Care Facility, and these are reflected in all Departments. Nursing in Extended Care is geared more toward rehabilitation (no matter how tedious the process), and also to long-term goals: the Dietary Department is usually planning a single menu for each special diet need (instead of offering choices of food only possible in Acute Facilities): the Activity Coordinator must work closely with Nursing so as to conflict as little as possible with routine care and treatments: the Activity Coordinator not only provides individual attention, but also sees that a Group Exercise Program for others is provided. Individual Physical and Speech Therapy can be ordered by the Physician, as well as some services of the Cardiopulmonary Dept. of the Acute Hospital.

Aside from the variance in physical set-up, nursing goals, Interdepartmental functions, etc., one finds a distinct difference in the personnel employed in the Extended Care Facility that meets its obligations successfully. There is an increased attitude of hopefulness, there is warmth, cheerfulness, an understanding and acceptance of the changes brought about by old age and illness, a desire to bring a measure of pleasure to others (no matter how transient), a sincere respect for the dignity of the elderly infirm, and above all, the gift of patience.

If the problems, frustrations, and habits of the elderly are repugnant, if one cannot easily accept the fact that old age with its frequently sad manifestations can be the lot of all of us, if one does not have a true desire to fully participate in this rewarding field of medicine, it is best to leave this area to others more qualified, and pursue a different course, not necessarily less meaningful, but more suitable.

8

Body Systems

EACH OF THE FOLLOWING SECTIONS provides basic information on how the body works. Many of the problems stroke and aphasic victims confront result from a breakdown in one or more of these "body systems." Our pressured physicians often do not have adequate time to describe what is going on in our body, or we are too distressed to remember. We can easily, with very few words, allay fear and apprehension when we ourselves have even scant knowledge.

SKELETAL SYSTEM

There are **206** bones in the human body which form the skeletal system. The femur is the longest of these bones. The bones are held together by ligaments at the joints. Muscles, which are se-

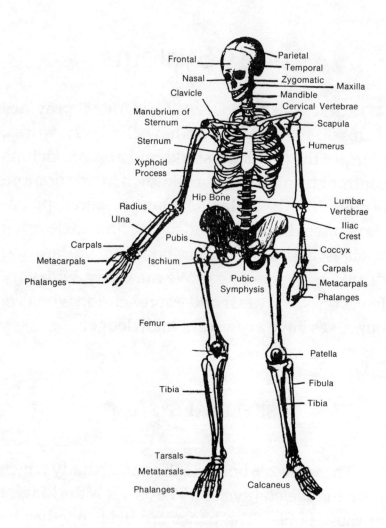

SKELETAL SYSTEM

cured to the bones by means of tendons, provide movement.

Bone is living tissue and is the hardest connective tissue serving to support the body. Bones are divided into four classes—long, short, flat, and irregular. Compact bone is the hard portion of the exterior, and cancellous (spongy) bone comprises the interior of the bone. Bone marrow, a jelly or sponge-like material, is found inside the bone. The main functions of the marrow are to manufacture red blood cells (erythrocytes), white blood cells (leukocytes), and platelets.

Bones are covered by periosteum, a very thin tissue which allows the blood supply to enter the bone. The periosteum also contains nerve structures. The cap of the end of the long bones is the epiphysis and the shaft is called the diaphysis. During the period of growth the epiphyses are separated from the main part of the bone by cartilage. Cartilage forms the major part of the bone in the very young and this allows for great flexibility. As the child grows, calcium phosphate appears in the cartilage, causing the bone to become harder.

The most common bone disorder is fracture. Some of the other disorders and diseases are osteitis (inflammation), Paget's disease (a disease characterized by progressive bowing and thickening of the shafts of the long bones—also called osteitis deformans), osteomalacia (softening of bone because of loss of calcium or from disease), rickets (a disturbance of ossification of bone due to Vitamin D deficiency), osteoporosis (softening due to atrophy—a common affliction of the elderly), periostitis (inflammation of the outer covering of the bone), Pott's disease (osteitis of the spine), primary as well as metastatic malignancies, and whiplash injury of the neck (compression of the cervical spine which involves the bones and intervertebral disks—usually caused by rear-end automobile collisions).

Operative procedures include the most common closed reduction of a fracture (manipulation and application of cast or splint), open reduction with internal fixation—ORIF (insertion of plate, screws, nails, or prosthesis), bone grafts, osteoclasis (surgical refracture of a bone because of malunion of fractured parts), osteoplasty (plastic surgery of the bones), osteotomy (the surgical cutting of a bone), amputation (the removal of a limb), and the newer, very effective total joint replacements.

Because of the high rate of successful reconstruction and therapy, thereby often allowing a return to normal or near normal activity, orthopedics—the science of prevention, diagnosis, and treatment of musculoskeletal diseases and abnormalities—is a rewarding field.

MUSCULAR SYSTEM

A muscle is an organ which produces movement when it contracts. There are three types of muscles— voluntary, involuntary, and cardiac.

Voluntary muscles are controlled by the conscious part of the brain. When we walk, write, or move about in any way we are using our voluntary muscles—in other words, these muscles move at our command. Unlike other body muscles, they are subject to fatigue with prolonged use.

Involuntary muscles are found in the muscular layer of the intestines, the blood vessels, bladder, organs of respiration, etc. These muscles of the alimentary tract and intestines produce peristalsis (a continuous worm-like movement which propels the contents along the tract). They work, as the name implies, without our conscious control, carrying on their duties automatically.

The cardiac muscle is also involuntary but is distinguished by a difference in the structure of its tissue. This muscle, of course, is in constant action during one's lifetime.

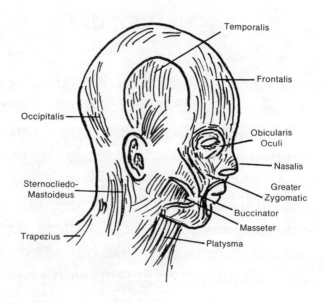

SOME MUSCLES OF THE HEAD

The voluntary muscles are striated or striped, the involuntary muscle tissue is described as un-striated or smooth, whereas the cardiac muscle is made up of striated fibers of a different type than the voluntary muscle fibers.

Muscles remain somewhat contracted at all times. This contraction or muscle tone (called tonus) serves to keep the body erect and the bones in their proper position. Muscle elasticity allows for the ability to stretch. Muscles can perform reflex action because they are served by both motor and sensory nerves. Muscular tissue of the three types comprises 40–50% of our body weight.

Muscles that allow a limb or joint to bend or flex are flexor muscles. Muscles that allow straightening are called extensor muscles. When movement is made away from the midline of the body, this is called abduction, and when move-ment is made toward the body it is described as adduction. (A "memory crutch" in this instance might be remembering that adduction means to *add to*, bring *toward*.)

A few of the conditions in which muscles are affected are: myositis (an inflammatory disease of the voluntary muscles), paralysis (resulting in loss of voluntary movements and sensation—temporary or permanent), torticollis (wryneck—caused by contraction of the cervical muscles, resulting in twisting of the neck), muscular dystrophy (a progressive disease causing extensive wasting away of muscles), myasthenia gravis (a chronic disease which also causes muscular weakness, most frequently affecting muscles of eyelids, throat, and face).

RESPIRATORY SYSTEM

The Respiratory System is clinically divided into two parts, the upper and lower. The upper respiratory organs are the nose, mouth, pharynx, larynx, and the trachea. The lower respiratory system consists of the bronchi, the lungs, the pleural spaces, and the thoracic cage. The diaphragm and intercostal muscles are also involved in the functioning of the lower respiratory system. The function of the respiratory system is to provide a means by which oxygen can be brought to the

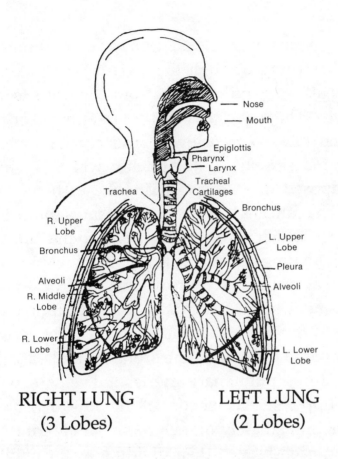

Nose

Mouth

Epiglottis
Pharynx
Larynx

Tracheal
Cartilages

Trachea

Bronchus

R. Upper
Lobe

L. Upper
Lobe

Bronchus

Pleura

Alveoli

Alveoli

R. Middle
Lobe

R. Lower
Lobe

L. Lower
Lobe

RIGHT LUNG
(3 Lobes)

LEFT LUNG
(2 Lobes)

body cells and carbon dioxide eliminated from the body.

The nose serves as a passage for receiving the air and also for eliminating the air after the oxygen has been removed in the lungs. The air is warmed, filtered (by hairs attached to the mucous membranes), and moistened in the nose. If the nasal passages are blocked, air can enter the lungs by breathing through the mouth. The pharynx (throat) transmits the air from the nose to the larynx. The larynx (or voice box) is situated on top of the trachea and below the root of the tongue. It terminates below in the trachea which is a tube composed of a series of ringlike cartilage and which branches into two main bronchi (bronchial tubes), which in turn carry the air to the lungs.

The lungs are the true organs of respiration. They are separated from one another by the heart and mediastinal structures. The right lung has 3 lobes (upper, middle, and lower). The left lung is composed of 2 lobes. The bronchus and vascular structures (pulmonary arteries and veins) enter at the upper surface or root of the lung. The bronchus immediately branches out on entering the lung, each branch then dividing again until finally they are expanded into small air sacs called alveoli. The actual exchange of air is accomplished through the alveoli, the oxygen entering and carbon dioxide being discharged. The exterior of the lungs is covered by a thin membrane called the pleura.

The diaphragm, a strong muscle separating the thoracic and abdominal cavities, flattens as it contracts during inhalation, thereby enlarging the chest cavity and allowing for expansion of the lungs.

Some respiratory diseases encountered in extended care facilities:

Chronic Pulmonary Emphysema: This is a lung disorder in which the terminal bronchioles become plugged with mucus, eventually resulting in loss of elasticity in the lung tissue also, so that breathing becomes difficult. This condition develops slowly over a period of years and is found most frequently in men over 40.

Bronchitis: Inflammation of the bronchi. Bronchitis can be either acute or chronic; an acute case occasionally develops into a chronic one. If the inflammation reaches the bronchioles and the alveoli, the condition is bronchopneumonia. Chronic bronchitis usually attacks the middle-aged and elderly, interfering with the air flow from the lungs, causing shortness of breath and constant coughing and expectoration.

Pleurisy: Inflammation of the pleura (the delicate membrane encasing the lung) which may be a complication of pneumonia, influenza, etc.

Pneumonia: Acute inflammation or infection of the lung.

Pulmonary Embolism: Usually a blood clot within the vascular system which obstructs the pulmonary artery. The clot is most often swept into circulation from a large peripheral vein, particularly one in the leg or pelvis. Plugging of a large pulmonary vessel can cause sudden death; however, in many cases anticoagulant drugs are used to aid in removal of the clot.

GASTROINTESTINAL SYSTEM

The Digestive System (alimentary canal) includes the mouth, teeth, tongue, pharynx, esophagus, stomach, and intestines. The entire canal from the mouth to the anus measures about 30 feet.

The mouth (also called the buccal cavity), the teeth, tongue, and jaws begin the process of digestion by masticating the food and combining it with saliva containing the enzyme ptyalin which begins to change the starches into sugar. When the food is then swallowed, the nasal passages and larynx are each sealed off momentarily by the soft palate and epiglottis, thereby allowing the food to pass into the esophagus and not into the trachea.

Peristalsis, the worm-like movement by which the muscles of the alimentary canal push the food along, allows the food to move through

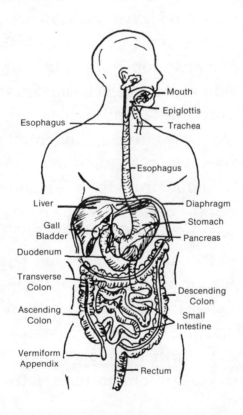

GASTROINTESTINAL SYSTEM

the esophagus to the stomach where the food is mixed and churned with the gastric juices (pepsin, lipase, and rennin), mucin, and hydrochloric acid, further breaking the mixture down to a form that the body can assimilate. The stomach of the average adult holds about 1½ quarts. A normal meal takes about 4 hours to be digested and to pass from the stomach to the small intestine.

When the food leaves the stomach it is a thick mixture called chyme which passes through the pylorus (the lower opening of the stomach) and enters the duodenum which is the first section of the small intestine (about 10" in length). The pancreatic juices flow into the duodenum which further break down protein, starch, and fat. The common bile duct from the gallbladder also discharges into the duodenum, the bile emulsifying the fat.

Below the duodenum is the jejunum (the longest portion of the small intestine) and the ileum which is the last and narrowest portion of the small intestine. As the food passes along these sections it is further broken down into usable substances (sugars, amino acids, fatty acids, and glycerin), which are easily absorbed through the lining of the small intestine.

The unusable parts of the food are passed on to the large intestine through the ileocecal valve which is the joining point of the ileum of the small intestine and cecum (the first portion of the large intestine). The veriform (meaning worm-shaped) appendix is attached to the cecum.

The large intestine from the cecum downward is divided into the ascending (moving upward), transverse (crosswise), and descending (downward) colon (these measure about 5½ feet altogether), and the sigmoid colon, which is the S-shaped bend at the distal end of the colon. The sigmoid colon then empties into the rectum. During its travels down the large intestine, liquid in the waste materials is absorbed through the walls of the large intestine and the bulky and useless materials are then emptied into the rectum and subsequently eliminated through the anus as stool or feces, the dark color of which is due to bile pigments.

The mechanism of the gastrointestinal tract has in this remarkable way served its purpose of utilizing the nutrients that are necessary to life and has eliminated those wastes that are of no value.

Some common gastrointestinal (G.I.) disorders encountered in geriatrics:

Ulcer: Gastric ulcer is an ulceration of the mucous membrane which lines the stomach. Duodenal ulcer is essentially the same type of ulceration but occurs in the duodenum. Bland diets are usually prescribed and also limitations on smoking and alcoholic intake. If untreated, an ulcer can perforate, causing bleeding and serious complications. **Colitis** is an inflammation of the colon which can lead to ulceration. In Extended Care Facilities we most often encounter spastic colitis, irritable colon, mucous colitis or functional bowel distress. Usually a bland diet is prescribed— strong seasonings, alcohol, coffee, etc. are excluded, also laxatives. **Gastritis** is an inflammation of the stomach. It can be either acute (caused by bacterial infection, food poisoning etc.) or chronic which occurs over a long period of time. Again, the patient is placed on a special diet, usually antacids are prescribed, and sometimes mild sedative or tranquilizer. **Diarrhea** is abnormal liquidity and frequency of fecal discharge, caused usually by infection or emotional disorders. Special diet and medication as indicated are usually prescribed. **Fecal impaction** is the condition of hardened feces in the rectum or sigmoid. When other means are not successful, the feces must be manually removed and changes in diet, medication, and increased fluid intake considered.

CARDIOVASCULAR SYSTEM
(CIRCULATORY)

The body's blood supply is contained in branched tubes called blood vessels and the action of the heart propels the blood through these tubes. The arteries are the vessels that conduct the blood out of the heart to body parts, while the veins bring the blood back to the heart. There is a network of very fine vessels, the capillaries, that allow the blood to circulate to tissues from the arteries in order to nourish them, and then back into the veins before returning to the heart. The Lymphatic System is an additional means of returning fluid from the tissues. The Circulatory

CARDIOVASCULAR SYSTEM

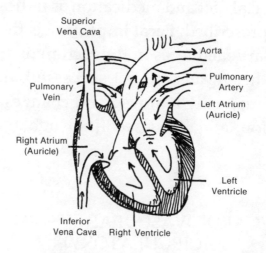

System, therefore, is concerned with the movement of blood and lymph.

The Vascular or Blood System is the main means of carrying nutriments and oxygen to the body cells. The average adult has about 5 quarts of blood, the entire amount normally circulating through the body every minute. Blood is composed of plasma (a pale yellow liquid) containing lymphocytes (white blood corpuscles), erythrocytes (red blood corpuscles), and thrombocytes (blood platelets). Arterial blood is bright red in color whereas venous blood becomes very dark or brownish-red before returning to the heart and lungs where it gets rid of its wastes and picks up a new supply of oxygen which turns the blood a bright red again.

Lymph is a transparent, slightly yellow liquid about 95% water, the remainder consisting of lymphocytes, plasma proteins, and other chemical substances. When tissue fluid from the blood plasma seeps through the capillary walls and is collected by the Lymphatic System, it is called lymph. When the lymph returns to the blood it again becomes plasma. Lymph nodes are lymphoid tissue which protect our body by filtering and destroying bacteria.

The heart is a hollow, hard-working organ (actually a pump) about the size of a fist. Its function is to pump the blood to the lungs and all the body tissues by way of the vascular and lymph systems as described above. The chambers of the heart are lined by a membrane called endocardium. The rough muscular wall surrounding the heart is the myocardium which in turn is covered by a fiber-like bag called the pericardium. A wall, or septum, divides the heart into right and left halves. Each side of the heart is then again divided, forming two upper chambers and two lower chambers. The upper chambers are the right and left atrium (sometimes called auricle), and the lower chambers are the right and left ventricle. Valves regulate the flow of blood through these four chambers and to the arteries. The right heart receives the dark red blood that has just returned after delivering its oxygen and nutrients. This blood is then pumped to the lungs where it rids itself of CO_2 and takes up oxygen again. It then is pumped into the left heart and sent from there through the large aorta to be distributed throughout the body.

Aside from the doctor's skill in detecting abnormalities by use of the stethoscope (in addition to observation and symptomatology of the patient), the electrocardiogram (ECG or EKG) is of great value in diagnosing many cardiac disorders such as abnormal rhythms, drug effects, etc. The electrocardiogram is a tracing of the small electrical impulses that the heart generates. The current accompanying the action of the heart is amplified many times, thereby moving a needle on a strip of paper so as to make a pattern of heart waves which can be measured and interpreted by the physician.

Some disorders of the heart:

Coronary insufficiency is a condition in which the coronary arteries are unable to transport adequate supply of oxygenated blood to nourish the heart muscle itself. One form of coronary insufficiency, **Angina Pectoris,** is often precipitated by hampered circulation of the blood caused by arteriosclerotic narrowing of the coronary artery. A **"heart attack"** is the common description for a condition in which the formation of a blood clot within a coronary artery may shut off (occlude) blood flow to a section of the heart muscle. This is called **Coronary Thrombosis** or occlusion. **Heart Failure** is inability of the heart to perform its function of pumping enough blood to assure a normal flow through the circulation. In **Congestive Heart Failure** one or more chambers of the heart do not empty sufficiently during contraction of the heart muscle, resulting in shortness of breath, edema (abnormal accumulation of fluid), weakness, and sometimes cyanosis and confusion in elderly patients. **Cardiac Arrhythmias** (abnormal rhythm of heart beat) are disturbances in the normal rate. The various forms of arrhythmia are sinus arrhythmia, extrasystole,

heart block, atrial fibrillation, paroxysmal tachy-
cardia and atrial flutter.

GENITOURINARY

The Genitourinary System deals with the organs in the production and excretion of urine, as
well as the male and female organs of reproduction, since anatomically they are so closely re-
lated.

The two kidneys, two ureters, bladder, and
urethra comprise the urinary system. The kidneys

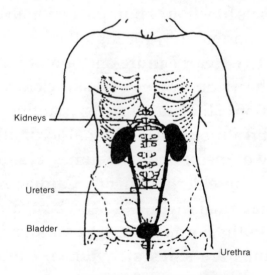

URINARY SYSTEM

are bean-shaped, glandular, filtering organs that regulate the amount of fluid and other substances in the blood, secreting urine which is water combined with various blood wastes. The blood enters the kidney by way of the renal artery, then is distributed into capillaries and nephrons. Nephrons are the basic unit of the kidney. There are about a million nephrons in each kidney and each works to produce urine.

The ureters (tubes about one foot long) conduct the urine to the urinary bladder from the kidneys by means of rhythmic contractions. The bladder is the hollow sac into which the urine drains from the ureters. It has muscular walls which expand and allow the urine to collect until voiding occurs, at which time the sphincters (circular muscles) where the bladder and urethra join, are relaxed and the urine is forced out. The urethra is the tube which extends from the bladder to the outside of the body. In the female the urethra is about 1½" long with its opening between the vagina and the clitoris. In the male the urethra is about 8" long and extends through the penis to the meatus (the opening at the tip of the penis).

The male pelvic or reproductive organs consist of the penis, the scrotum (two skin covered pouch-like sacs divided by a septum or partition), the two testes (the singular for this word is testis) which are egg-shaped glands situated in the scrotum and suspended by the spermatic cords, the epididymis which is a long cord-like structure along the border of the testis which stores the sperm, the vas deferens (also called ductus deferens) which joins the excretory duct of the seminal vesicles—two membranous pouches placed between the bladder and the rectum—to form the ejaculatory duct. The ejaculatory ducts pass through the prostate gland which produces a thin fluid that flows into the urethra through the ducts. The prostate is a muscular gland with three lobes and the normal gland is about the size of a walnut.

The female glands of reproduction consist of two ovaries (the sex glands, or gonads, in which the ova or seeds are formed, and which also produce essential hormones), the fallopian tubes which attach to the ovaries by means of fringe-like processes (fimbriae), the uterus (the hollow muscular organ in which the fetus grows), the vagina (the canal from the external genitalia to the cervix or neck of the uterus which receives the penis as it discharges spermatozoa during coitus—intercourse), the external genitalia and the breasts. The ovum which is produced in the ovaries passes through the fallopian tubes to the uterus where it is either impregnated by spermatozoa or disintegrates and is discharged. Occasionally an ovum is impregnated in the tube before reaching the uterus (ectopic pregnancy), in which case surgical intervention is usually necessary.

The uterus, which is normally about the size of a pear, consists of the fundus (upper portion), the body (middle portion), and the cervix (lower portion or neck). The muscular lining of the uterus is the myometrium and the inner lining is called the endometrium. The myometrial tissues go through the monthly cycle of growth and discharge (menstruation); however, in the event of a fertilized egg, the tissues are utilized by the embryo and no menstruation occurs.

NERVOUS SYSTEM

The Nervous System provides us with consciousness of our existence and the ability to make
adjustments of function. Its anatomy is extremely
complicated and we can cover a very few high-
lights in this brief study, hopefully enough so that
the reader will have at least a minimal background from which to pursue study.

The Nervous System is divided both anatomically and functionally into the brain, the spinal
cord, and the nerves. The brain and the spinal
cord comprise the CENTRAL NERVOUS SYSTEM
(C.N.S.), and the series of nerves that reach from
the C.N.S. to all body parts is designated as the
PERIPHERAL NERVOUS SYSTEM. The peripheral
nervous system itself is divided into the Auto-
nomic System (operates without our conscious
control—automatically—i.e., heart and glands),
and the Voluntary System (controls muscles and
carries information to the brain).

The functional unit of the nervous system is
the nerve cell, or neuron. It is a cord-like structure
which conveys impulses from the C.N.S. to another region of the body. Like other cells of the

body it has a nucleus surrounded by cytoplasm. The neuron possesses irritability which makes it capable of stimulation, and it is also capable of conducting impulses. When groups of these cells are outside the brain or spinal cord they are called ganglia; however, when they are in the brain or spinal cord, they are called nuclei. Nerves are classified as sensory, motor, or mixed. Sensory nerves carry information to the brain—i.e. pain, heat, or cold. Motor nerves serve to transmit impulses from the brain and spinal cord to the muscles. Mixed nerves have both motor and sensory fibers and are capable of sending messages in both directions.

The brain is a mass of pinkish-gray tissue contained within the cranium and weighing about three pounds. It consists of the **cerebrum** (the largest portion, which is the thinking and reasoning center and also receives information from the senses and directs movement of the body), the **cerebellum** (controls balance and coordination of muscles), the **medulla oblongata** (a very vital part of the brain since it controls the involuntary movements of the heart and breathing mechanism), and the **pons varolii** which lies

THE BRAIN

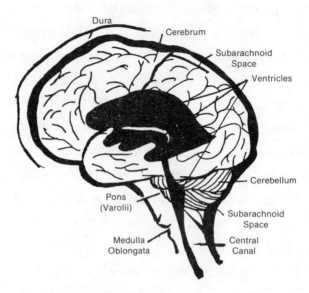

in front of the cerebrum and serves as a bridge between the medulla and cerebellum. There are twelve cranial nerves attached to the brain, one nerve of each pair lying on each side of the head.

The spinal cord is protected by the vertebrae as it passes through its central portions. It consists of nerve fibers that pass to and away from the brain. Thirty-one pairs of spinal nerves are given off from the spinal cord, one on each side leading to other parts of the body. Both the brain and spinal cord are covered by three protective membranes—the dura mater, arachnoid, and pia mater. The cerebrospinal fluid which runs through the spinal cord and ventricles of the brain protects the soft structures of the Central Nervous System.

Some diseases of the nervous system are brain abscess, brain tumor, cerebral hemorrhage (rupture of a cerebral vessel), cerebral palsy, cerebral thrombosis, encephalitis, epilepsy, hydrocephalus (abnormal accumulation of fluid in the brain), meningitis (inflammation of the meninges), multiple sclerosis (a disease characterized by hardened patches scattered throughout the brain and spinal cord which interfere with the nerve function), myelitis (inflammation of the spinal cord), Parkinson's disease or paralysis agitans (a disorder of the brain stem resulting in tremors, slow motion, etc.), poliomyelitis (a viral disease with lesions in the Central Nervous System), subdural hematoma (a blood tumor caused by bleeding into the subdural space), and tabes dorsalis (syphilis of the Central Nervous System).

Some signs and symptoms of nervous system disease are tremors, convulsions, paralysis, lack of coordination, headache due to pressure within the cranial cavity, projectile vomiting, etc. It must be understood, however, that many of these symptoms can also be due to other than nervous system pathology.

Organic Brain Syndrome is a common disorder of the elderly. These syndromes are mental disorders usually caused by impaired cerebral tissue function. Organic brain syndrome can be either acute brain syndrome, a transient condition, or chronic brain syndrome, damage irreversible. The patient with organic brain syndrome will show impairment in one or several areas—memory, reduced attention span, impairment in comprehension and judgement and exaggerated emotional responses. Psychoses can be associated with organic brain syndrome attributed to many things. Presenile dementias appear in patients under 60 years of age. Psychoses may also be caused by cerebral arteriosclerosis, cerebrovascular disturbances such as hypertension and heart disease, etc. It is important to the patient to be in familiar surroundings and to participate in activities that he is capable of performing. Tranquilizers are often used for the agitated patient and antidepressants as indicated. Alzheimer's Disease is a presenile dementia which has become more commonly recognized in recent years.

ENDOCRINE SYSTEM

The Endocrine System is comprised of ductless glands, meaning glands that produce secretions that are absorbed into the blood stream by the capillary blood vessels and lymphatics that course through them, rather than being poured through ducts into some other part of the body, as is true of the gastrointestinal system. These secretions are called **hormones** and they are of extreme importance to the body, as is evidenced by the maladies that affect us when the glands are either over or under secreting. There is still much to be learned regarding all the functions of the ductless glands, and in our very simplified study we will attempt to discuss only the high points.

The endocrine glands are the **pituitary, thyroid, parathyroids, islets of Langerhans** in the pancreas, **adrenals, testes,** and **ovaries.** The **pineal** (located in the center part of the brain) and the **thymus** (located at the upper part of the sternum) are also classified as endocrine glands.

The **thyroid** gland is situated in the neck and has two lobes, one on each side of the larynx with a small middle lobe called the isthmus. The hormone it secretes is thyroxin (containing up to 65% iodine) which controls metabolism, the vital life activity of all the body cells. If the gland is over-active (hyperactive) a person feels flushed and warmer than ordinary, requires less clothing, per-spires easily, has a rapid pulse, eats in excess but at the same time loses weight and generally

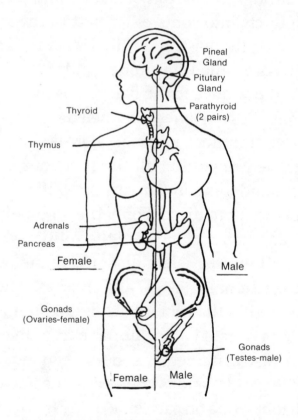

THE ENDOCRINE GLANDS

shows the effects of high metabolism. Hyperthyroidism can produce Graves' disease or exophthalmic goiter (thus named because of the characteristic protruding of the eyeballs). If the gland is underactive (hypoactive) there is a disturbance of the water balance and the person is easily fatigued, runs a subnormal temperature, and gains weight. If this condition is severe and is not corrected in childhood, the resulting underdevelopment and retardation is called cretinism. If the condition occurs in adulthood, is severe and untreated, the disease is called myxedema.

The **parathyroid** glands are actually two pairs of small glands at the base or back portion of the thyroid gland. They secrete parathyroid hormone which regulates the blood calcium level. Over-secretion (hyperparathyroidism), which is usually caused by a benign tumor (adenoma), can result in large bone cysts or even in pathologic fractures. Under-secretion (hypoparathyroidism), which can be caused by injury to the parathyroids, can cause tetany (a continuous spasm of a muscle).

The **islets of Langerhans** are very specialized cells scattered throughout the pancreas. They produce the hormone insulin which is essential to proper carbohydrate utilization. Lack of insulin causes diabetes mellitus.

The **adrenal** glands are located one on top of each kidney. Each is made up of a cortex and a medulla, both parts secreting different substances, to a total of at least 26 hormones. The cortex produces hormones which increase blood sodium and sugar, decrease blood potassium, and govern certain secondary sex characteristics. The medulla produces the hormone epinephrine (adrenalin) which elevates blood pressure, increases muscle energy, and increases the heartbeat.

The **ovaries** produce the hormones estrogen and progesterone, both of which stimulate the development of secondary female sex characteristics and also affect the endometrium (lining of the uterus).

The **testes** produce testosterone which stimulates the development of secondary male characteristics and is necessary for normal functioning of the male reproductive organs.

ORGANS OF SPECIAL SENSE

The organs of sense are taste, smell, sight, and hearing. The general sensations of heat, cold, pain, and pressure can also be classified as organs of special sense.

TASTE: Taste is the sensation caused by contact of substances with the tongue. The taste buds are the organs of taste. These are cells which form papillae (projections) on various places on the tongue. There are four basic tastes—sweet, sour, salt, and bitter. Alkaline and metallic tastes are sometimes also included. Each taste bud is specialized and responds only to its particular basic taste.

SMELL: The organ of smell is known as the olfactory organ. It consists of the external nose and the internal or nasal cavities. There is a small pea-sized area inside each nasal cavity where the endings of the nerves of smell are located. The olfactory nerve is the first cranial nerve which carries the sense of smell to the brain where it is interpreted.

SIGHT: The eye is the organ of vision. It is a very delicate organ and is protected by the skull bones, the conjunctiva which covers the front of the eyeball and also lines the upper and lower eyelids. The lids and eyelashes also protect the eye as does the lacrimal duct which exudes tears that can wash the eye of foreign bodies. Light passes from the exterior through the cornea which is a transparent tissue in the front portion of the eye. The light then passes through the pupil and lens and through the watery or vitreous material which fills the eyeball, and then rests upon the retina. The retina contains many small nerve cells which conduct the light sensation to the brain where it is interpreted.

HEARING: The ear is the organ of hearing and also of equilibrium (balance). It is composed by an outer ear (external), middle ear, and inner ear (internal). The outer ear consists of the pinna (the projecting part of the ear lying outside the head) which picks up the sound waves and sends them to the acoustic meatus (passage leading to eardrum—tympanic membrane) which separates the outer from the middle ear. The middle ear contains 3 ossicles (small bones) called malleus (hammer), incus (anvil), and stapes (stirrup) since they resemble these objects in shape. The middle ear is also connected to the nasopharynx by way of the eustachian tube which serves to equalize the air pressure on both sides of the eardrum.

9

Understanding Nuclear Medicine and Diagnostic Procedures

TO THE PATIENT, AND OFTEN the medical worker as well, there is an aura of mystery and apprehension surrounding the term NUCLEAR MEDICINE. Granted, except for those very few individuals directly engaged in the field, we do not in any way fully understand the scientific research that led to the development of nuclear reactors as part of the atomic weapons program with its subsequent by-product of radioisotopes. It is indeed not at all necessary that we comprehend the mechanism and details. What *is* important is that we are well enough informed to be able to ease the usual anxiety (commonly recognized as "fear of the unknown") in our patients whenever these procedures are recommended by the physician.

Primarily, as medical and paramedical workers, we must be aware of the fact that Nuclear

Medicine procedures are painless, unless one finds it difficult to tolerate the pinprick of the simple intravenous injection which precedes the scan. This injection is of a specific radioactive material which concentrates in the organ or gland under suspicion. Following this, the patient is subjected only to occasional repositioning as the technician manipulates and controls the machine which produces the pictures or "scans" that are later interpreted by the physician specialist trained in Nuclear Medicine.

Nuclear Medicine is not a new field. In the past few years it has become more and more a significant diagnostic tool, causing an increasing awareness of it. It has been tried and proven to be a *safe* procedure. In fact, body radiation to the patient is recorded as less than emitted by a routine chest x-ray.

There has been tremendous progress in Nuclear Medicine in recent years, perhaps more than in any other field of medicine. It has become extremely important (often excelling x-ray procedures) in diagnosing many types of pathology—i.e. brain tumors, hematomas, arteriovenous malformations, and cerebrovascular disease. The lung scan is useful in diagnosing pulmonary embolism, thoracic tumors, and chronic obstructive lung disease. A spleen scan will show the spleen size, evidence of rupture, abscess, or cyst. Bone scans are of importance in detecting malignant tumors, metastatic carcinoma, as well as non-malignant lesions. The liver scan reveals hepatic size and shape and is used in diagnosing tumors, cysts, rupture, cirrhosis, and cancer metastasis.

The thyroid scan is unique in its ability to diagnose adenomas, carcinomas, or cysts. Radio-iodine therapy is of value in treating hyperthyroidism as well as thyroid cancer, often eliminating the need for surgical intervention.

There is also a newer diagnostic device, Magnetic Resonance Imaging (M.R.I.), which is considered to be a very safe and accurate procedure. The equipment operates without the use of any ionizing radiation and operates instead with the use of a magnetic field and varying radio-frequency energies.

Part III

Understanding
Medical Terminology

Medical Abbreviations
Prefixes
Roots
Suffixes

10

Medical Terminology

UNDERSTANDING MEDICAL TERMINOLOGY is quite important in learning to cope with any illness. There are, or course, many more word components in medical terminology than those presented here.

It doesn't take too much study of prefixes, roots, and suffixes to remove much of the "mystery" from medical terms. You probably knew at least some of the combinations without really realizing it. Since you understand "thyroid," and recognize that "itis" means inflammation, you can easily understand "thyroiditis." The same is true of "bronchitis," "apppendicitis," "tonsillitis," etc. Relate "ectomy" (removal, excision of an organ or part) to "appendectomy," "tonsillectomy," "thyroidectomy." When we learn that the prefix "hyper" means "over or excessive" you can easily understand "hyperthyroidism," "hyperventilation," etc. Now when you know that "myo" means muscle, you understand "myospasm," "myolipoma," and "myocarditis." We will learn that "peri" means around (like perimeter), that "cardi" refers to heart, that "itis" means inflammation. Putting all together we come up with "pericarditis" which translates to inflammation of the pericardium (the sac that surrounds the heart).

Because a word is *long* does not mean that you will have difficulty with it. Very soon, with very little reference to the dictionary, you will understand such long words as "gastroduodenoenterostomy" and "hysterosalpingo-oophorectomy!" An added bonus is that you will find pride in pronouncing medical terms correctly. TRY IT!

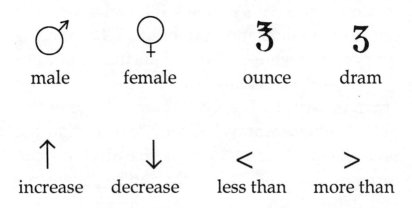

male   female   ounce   dram

increase   decrease   less than   more than

COMMON MEDICAL ABBREVIATIONS
(examples)

NOTE: In comparing several medical references, one finds slight differences in abbreviations, capitalization, and punctuation; however, those listed below are some of the most commonly used, although one can still encounter variances in many facilities.

abd—abdomen
a.c.—before meals
A.D.L.—activities of daily living
ad lib—at pleasure
A&P—anterior and posterior
b.i.d.—twice daily
BM—bowel movement
B.M.R.—basal metabolic rate
B.P.—blood pressure
BPH—benign prostatic hypertrophy
c̄—with
CAT—computerized axial tomography
c.b.c.—complete blood count
CBS—chronic brain syndrome
cc.—cubic centimeter
C.C.—Chief Complaint
cm.—centimeter
C.N.S.—central nervous system
C/O—complains of
COPD—chronic obstructive pulmonary disease
CPR—cardiopulmonary resuscitation
CVA—cerebrovascular accident (stroke)
DTR—deep tendon reflexes
EEG—electroencephalogram
E.E.N.T.—eye, ear, nose, throat

EKG. or ECG.—electrocardiogram
FB—foreign body
Fx—fracture
F.U.O.—fever of undetermined origin
GB—gallbladder
GI—gastrointestinal
gr.—grain
Gm.—gram
gt.—drop
gtt.—drops
GU—genitourinary
HCT.—hematocrit
HCVD—hypertensive cardiovascular disease
H.E.E.N.T.—Head, eye, ear, nose, and throat
Hgb.—hemoglobin
h.s.—at bedtime (hour of sleep)
HTN—hypertension
I & D—incision and drainage
I.M.—intramuscular
I and O—intake and output
IPPB.—intermittent positive pressure breathing
I.V.—intravenous
IVP.—intravenous pyelogram
K.—potassium (KCl. - potassium chloride)
k.j.—knee jerk
K.U.B.—kidney, ureter, and bladder
kg.—kilogram
Lat.—lateral
LP—lumbar puncture
m.—meter
mEq.—milliequivalent
mg.—milligram
mcg.—microgram
MI—myocardial infarction
ml.—milliliter

M.M.—mucous membranes
mm.—millimeter
M.R.I.—Magnetic Resonance Imaging
N.P.O.—nothing by mouth
O_2—oxygen
OBS—organic brain syndrome
O.D.—right eye
ORIF—open reduction internal fixation
O.S.—left eye
O.T.—Occupational Therapy
O.U.—both eyes
P&A—percussion and auscultation
p.c.—after meals
PDR—Physician's Desk Reference (drugs)
P.E.—physical examination
P.H.—Past History
P.M.I.—point of maximal impulse
P.O.—by mouth
p.r.n.—as circumstances may require
P.T.—Physical Therapy
q.—every
q. AM—every morning
q.d.—every day
q.h.—every hour (° for hour)
q.i.d.—4 times per day
q.s.—sufficient quantity
ROM—range of motion
s̄—without
ss —one half
SOB—shortness of breath
S.R.—sedimentation rate
Stat.—immediately
TIA—transient ischemic attack
t.i.d.—three times per day
TPR—temperature, pulse, and respirations

TURP—transurethral resection of prostate
ung.—ointment
URTI—upper respiratory tract infection
UTI—urinary tract infection
wt.—weight

PREFIXES

PREFIX	EXAMPLE	MEANING
AB- from, away	abnormal ab/normal	away from normal
A- AN- without, not	analgesia an/algesia	absence of pain
AD- increase, toward	adductor ad/ductor	drawing toward center
ANTE- before	anterior ante/rior	in front of
ANTI- against	antiseptic anti/septic	preventing infection
BI- two, twice	bilateral bi/lateral	affecting both sides
BRADY- slow	bradycardia brady/cardia	slow heart beat
CO- CON- together, with	congenital defect con/genital	born with a defect
CONTRA- against, opposite	contraindication contra/indication	undesirable to treatment
DIS- separation	dislocate dis/locate	displacement of a bone
DYS- difficult, painful	dysuria dys/uria	painful urination

PREFIX	EXAMPLE	MEANING
EC- EX- outside, away from	exhale ex/hale	breathe out
ENDO- within, inside	endocardium endo/cardium	membrane lining heart
EPI- on, upon	epidermis epi/dermis	top layer of skin
EXTRA- outside of	extravascular extra/vascular	situated outside a vessel
HEMI- one-half	hemiplegia hemi/plegia	paralysis one side of body
HYPER- over, excessive	hypertension hyper/tension	high blood pressure
HYPO- lack, beneath	hypoglycemia hypo/glycemia	low blood sugar
INFRA- below	inframaxillary infra/maxillary	situated beneath the jaw
INTRA- within	intrabuccal intra/buccal	within mouth or cheek
MEGA- large	megacolon mega/colon	abnormally large colon
META- change	metamorphosis meta/morphosis	change of shape

PREFIX	EXAMPLE	MEANING
ORTHO- straight, normal	orthodontics ortho/dontics	straightening of teeth
PACHY- thick	pachyderma pachy/derma	abnormal thickness of skin
PARA- beside	pararectal para/rectal	beside the rectum
PERI- around	pericardium peri/cardium	membrane around the heart
PRE- in front, before	presenility pre/senility	premature old age
PRO- forward, before	promontory pro/montory	projecting eminence, process
RETRO- backward, behind	retroversion retro/version	tipping of an organ backward
SAPRO- putrid	saprogenic sapro/genic	causing putrefaction
SUB- under, below	substernal sub/sternal	situated beneath sternum
SUPRA- SUPER- above, over	suprapatellar supra/patellar	situated above the patella
SYN- SYM- together, with	syndrome syn/drome	set of symptoms occurring together

PREFIX	EXAMPLE	MEANING
TOX- TOXI- poison	toxemia tox/emia	toxic products in blood
TRANS- across, through	transurethral trans/urethral	performed through the urethra
UNI- one	unilateral uni/lateral	affecting one side

ROOTS

ROOT	EXAMPLE	MEANING
ADEN- gland	adenoma aden/oma	glandular tissue tumor
AER- air	aerated aer/ated	filled with air
ANGI- vessel	angioma angi/oma	a tumor of blood vessels
ARTHR- joint	arthritis arth/ritis	inflammation of joints
BLEPHAR- eyelid	blepharitis blephar/itis	inflammation of eyelid
CARDI- heart	cardiovascular cardio/vascular	pertaining to heart & vessels
CEPHAL- head	cephalgia cephal/gia	headache
CEREBR- (CEREBRAL-) brain	cerebrospinal cerebro/spinal	pertaining to brain & spinal cord
CERVIC- neck	cervical cerv/ical	pertaining to the neck
CHEIL- lip	cheiloplasty cheilo/plasty	plastic operation of lip

ROOT	EXAMPLE	MEANING
CHIR- hand	chiromegaly chiro/megaly	abnormally large hands
CHOL(E)- pertaining to bile	cholecystitis chole/cystitis	inflammation of gallbladder
CHONDR- cartilage	chondromalacia chondro/malacia	softening of the cartilage
COST- rib	costochondral costo/chondral	pertaining to rib & cartilage
CRANIO- skull	craniotomy cranio/tomy	surgical opening of skull
CYST- bladder	cystoscope cysto/scope	instrument for exam. of bladder
CYT- cell	cytology cyt/ology	study of cell life
DACRY- tear	dacryorrhea dacry/orrhea	profuse flow of tears
DERMA- DERMAT- skin	dermatitis derma/titis	inflammation of the skin
ENCEPHAL- brain	encephalitis encephal/itis	inflammation of brain
ENTER- intestine	enteritis enter/itis	inflammation of intestines

ROOT	EXAMPLE	MEANING
GASTR- stomach	gastritis gastr/itis	inflammation of stomach
GLOSS- tongue	glossoplegia glosso/plegia	paralysis of the tongue
GLYC- sugar	glycosuria glyco/suria	sugar in the urine
HEM- blood	hematemesis hema/temesis	vomiting of blood
HEPAT- liver	hepatitis hepat/itis	inflammation of the liver
HYSTER- uterus	hysterectomy hyster/ectomy	surgical excision of the uterus
ILI- ilium	ilium ili/um	upper part of the hip bone
LEUC-, LEUK- white	leukopenia leuko/penia	abnormal decrease in white blood cells
LIP- fat	lipoma lip/oma	a fatty tumor
LITH- stone	lithiasis lith/iasis	presence of stones (kidney, gall bladder, etc.
MAST- breast	mastectomy mast/ectomy	surgical removal of breast

ROOT	EXAMPLE	MEANING
MENING- membrane	meningitis menin/gitis	inflammation membrane cord/brain
METR- uterus	metrorrhagia metro/rrhagia	bleeding from uterus
MY-, MYO- muscle	myocardium myo/cardium	layer heart wall (cardiac muscle)
NEPHR- kidney	nephrosis neph/rosis	disease of the kidney
OPHTHALM- eye	ophthalmology ophthalm/ology	study of eye and its diseases
OSTEO- bone	osteomyelitis osteo/myelitis	inflammation of bone
PNEUM- lung	pneumothorax pneumo/thorax	accumulation of air in pleural cavity
PROCT- rectum	proctoscope procto/scope	instrument to inspect rectum
PSYCH- mind, soul	psychotherapy psycho/therapy	treatment by mental affects
PYEL- pelvis, kidney	pyelitis pyel/itis	inflammation of pelvis of kidney

ROOT	EXAMPLE	MEANING
PYLOR- pylorus (opening of stomach to duodenum)	pylorospasm pyloro/spasm	spasm of the pylorus
PYO- pus	pyorrhea pyo/rrhea	inflammation/ pus from gums
SPONDYL- vertebra	spondylolithesis spondylo/ lithesis	forward displacement of vertebra
TEST- testis (male gonad)	testicular test/icular	pertaining to a testis (pl. testes)
TRACHE- tube from larynx to bronchi	tracheitis trache/itis	inflammation of the trachea
VISC(ERO)- organ of body	visceral visc/eral	pertaining to internal organs

SUFFIXES

SUFFIX	EXAMPLE	MEANING
-ALGIA pain	neuralgia neur/algia	pain along course of nerves
-CELE hernia	cystocele cysto/cele	herniation of urinary bladder into the vagina
-CENTESIS puncture	paracentesis para/centesis	surgical puncture and drainage of a cavity
-ECTOMY excision organ	tonsillectomy tonsill/ectomy	removal of tonsils
-EMIA blood condition	hyperglycemia hyperglyc/emia	high blood sugar
-GENIC to produce	pathogenic patho/genic	produces disease
-ITIS inflammation	cystitis cyst/itis	inflammation urinary bladder
-LYSIS to free, release	hemolysis hemo/lysis	liberation of hemoglobin
-MEGALY enlargement	hepatomegaly hepato/megaly	enlargement of liver
-OMA tumor	adenoma aden/oma	glandular tumor

SUFFIX	EXAMPLE	MEANING
-OSIS condition	arteriosclerosis arterioscler/osis	hardening of the arteries
-PATHY disease	adenopathy adeno/pathy	disease of a gland
-PENIA decrease	leukopenia leuko/penia	decrease leuko- cytes of blood
-PEXY fixation	nephropexy nephro/pexy	fixation of a kidney
-PLASTY surgical repair	arthroplasty arthro/plasty	plastic surgery of a joint
-PTOSIS prolapse, droop	bletharoptosis bletharo/ptosis	drooping of eyelid
-RRHAGE (RRHAGIA) excessive flow	hemorrhage hemo/rrhage	copious escape of blood
-RRHAPHY repair	herniorrhaphy hernio/rrhaphy	repair of a hernia
-RRHEA flow, discharge	diarrhea dia/rrhea	too frequent fecal discharge
-SCOPY inspect	cystoscopy cysto/scopy	inspect bladder with instrument
-STOMY surgical opening between two structures	colostomy colo/stomy	surgical opening of colon to body surface

SUFFIX	EXAMPLE	MEANING
-TOMY incision into	thoracotomy thoraco/tomy	surgical opening of chest
-TRIPSY crushing	lithotripsy litho/tripsy	crushing of stone in bladder

PART IV

BASIC NEEDS ILLUSTRATIONS
Pain/Itch
Thirsty
Hungry
Turn over
Bed up/down
Bedpan
Urinal
Toilet
Too hot
Too cold
Light off/on
Brush teeth

11

Basic Needs Illustrations

THE IMPORTANCE OF BASIC NEEDS ILLUSTRA-
TIONS has been previously mentioned. There
are some aphasic patients who are capable of
recognizing and responding to pictures, either by
reading or pointing, or sometimes by changes in
facial expressions, so that these needs can be
known.

Following is a demonstration of the illustrations that could be useful. It is stressed, however,
that nurses, home health aids, family, and friends
could supplement by newspaper/magazine clip-
pings, or in any other way appropriate to the
individual need.

pain/ itch

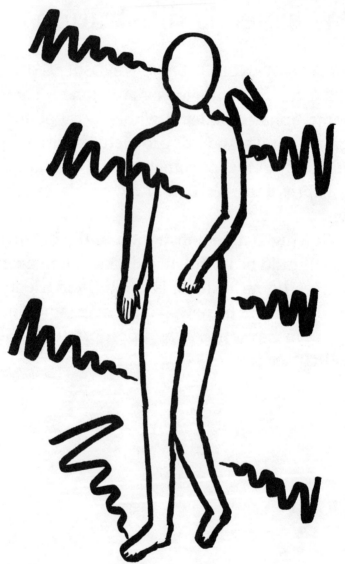

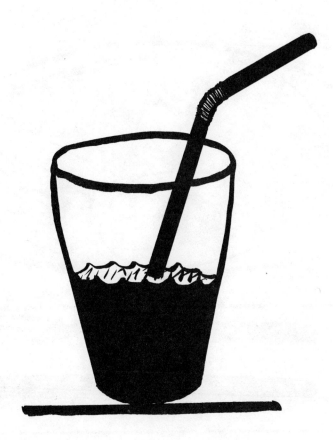

thirsty

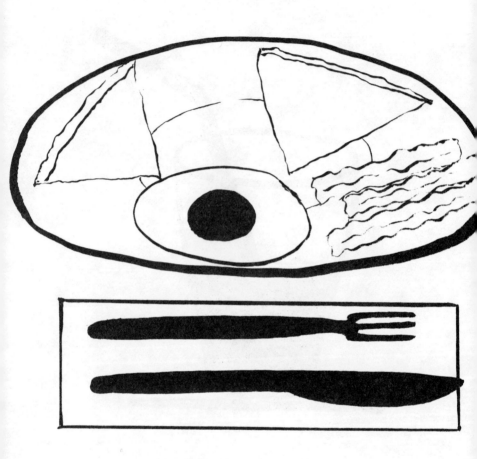

hungry

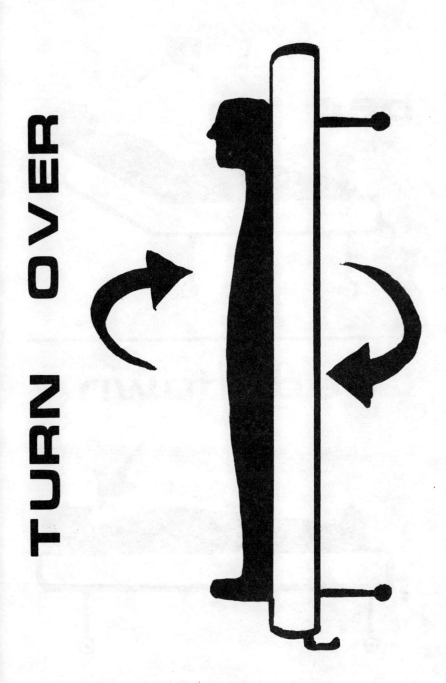

bed up

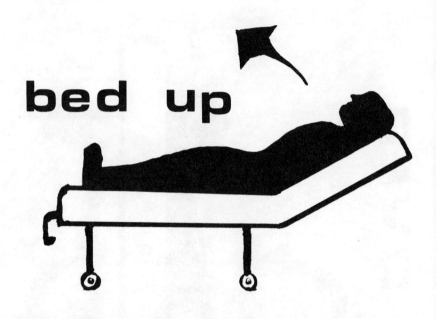

bed down

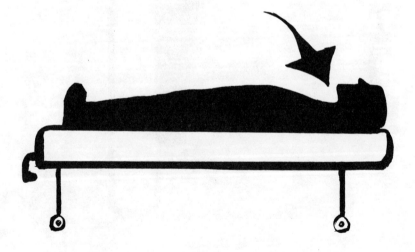

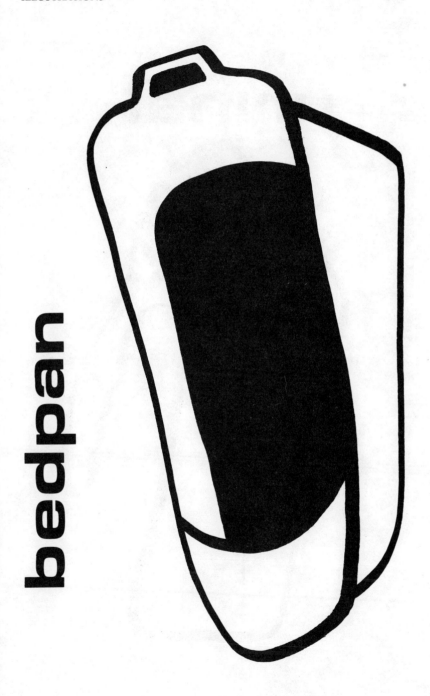

bedpan

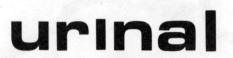

urinal

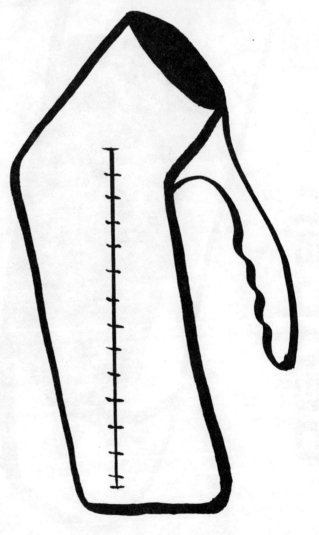

TOILET

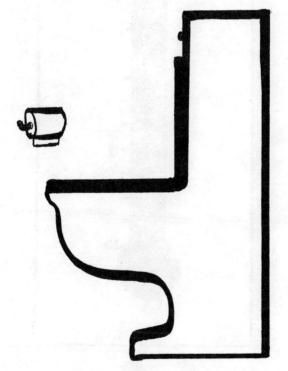

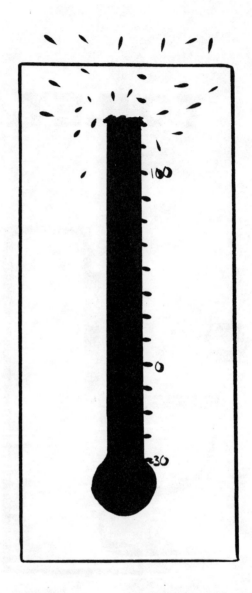

too hot

too cold

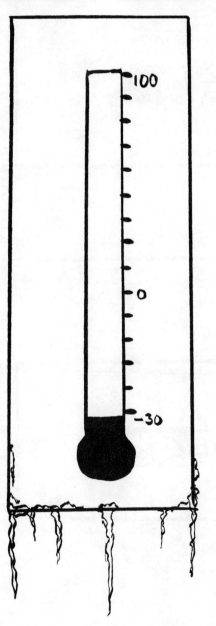

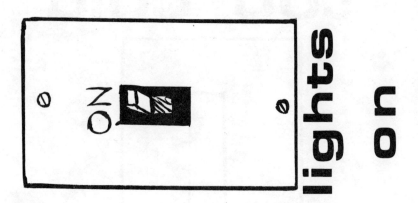

lights on

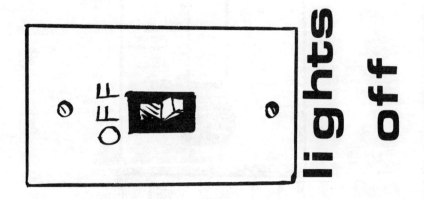

lights off

BRUSH TEETH

About the Author

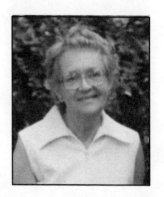

Helen Underwood was born in Berkeley, California in 1914, and has had a long and rewarding career serving others. Her interest in pursuing nursing as a career started with the terminal illness of her father who died of multiple sclerosis after several years of incapacity. Later she cared for her mother who suffered a severe stroke with aphasia.

After one year at the University of California, Berkeley, she began nurses' training at the UC Hospital in San Francisco, graduating as a Registered Nurse. After several years of private duty and office nursing, she enlisted in the Army Nurse Corps (1943) at the San Francisco Presidio as a Hospital Train Duty Nurse. From there she travelled all over the country delivering patients from the Pacific War area nearer their homes after initial care at the Presidio.

In 1944, she married Donald E. Underwood, an attorney. After losing twins in 1948, they adopted a male infant in 1949, and a seven-year-old boy nine years later.

Helen has taken many courses in teaching and has certified scores of nursing assistants in long-term care. She emphasizes understanding the problems and frustrations faced by elderly and terminal patients. "Only by knowing the symptoms and problems can one fully relate, sympathize, and properly care for the disabled." She hopes that nurses and family caregivers will benefit from her experience and suggestions.

Retired now, she makes her home in Grass Valley, California, and admits to needing, from time to time, a little bit of help herself.